THE SLEEP EASY SOLUTION BOOK

HOW TO STOP SLEEP APNEA, SNORING, AND SLEEP DISORDERS

Dr. Robertino Bedenian

THANK YOU!

First of all, I would like to thank you for choosing this e-book. The creation of this e-book is connected with the sincere desire to provide solid answers to questions on the subject of "sleep apnea and sleep disorders". During conversations, also within my circle of acquaintances and friends, it turned out that several questions are discussed time and again - sometimes controversially - when it comes to sleep apnea and sleep disorders. I also suffered from massive sleep disorders over a long period, which moved me to take a closer look at the causes of sleep disorders and, above all, to name suitable therapy options. Against this background, this e-book was created to answer questions about "sleep apnea and sleep disorders" in a simple and understandable form.

Before the issues surrounding the topic of "sleep apnea" are discussed in detail below, this term should first be briefly explained: Sleep apnea is a condition in which one stops breathing either temporarily or even completely during sleep. The breaths become progressively shallower before they stop completely. This state can last from a few seconds to even a few minutes. Sleep studies have shown that breathing cessations can even occur more than 30 times in 60 minutes. Pathological cessations of breathing last longer than ten seconds, causing the oxygen content of the blood to drop (hypoxemia). This leads to a deficiency in the supply of oxygen to the tissues and, as a result, there is an awakening reaction of the body, due to which breathing resumes. After that, the affected person breathes normally again. Sleep apnea is often accompanied by loud snoring. Sometimes the affected person appears as if he or she is suffocating for a brief moment: he or she gasps for air after the waking reaction has been triggered by the respiratory arrest. However, this "gasping for air" can also occur during sleep, i.e., the affected person does not necessarily have to wake up.

The symptoms will be discussed in detail in the next chapter.

The ongoing interruption of breathing naturally means that people do not get the restful sleep they desperately need at night. As a result, they feel tired and sleepy during the day. Although this will be discussed in detail in the following chapters, it should be noted at this point that it will not be easy to diagnose this condition. As a rule, the general practitioner will not be able to diagnose "sleep apnea" during a regular examination. Since this condition is only noticeable during sleep, those people who suffer from sleep apnea themselves are often unaware that they suffer from these symptoms. Usually, other people notice this unusual sleep pattern, and they need to make those people affected aware of it. However, in many cases, even then they might still not realize that these symptoms are due to "sleep apnea".

Millions of adults suffer from sleep apnea and don't even know it. The majority of them are overweight or obese. Men suffer from this condition more than women. The older a person, the more likely this condition might occur during sleep. In women, sleep apnea may develop after menopause. Groups of people, such as African Americans, South Americans, and Pacific Islanders, are found to have sleep apnea more often than other groups. Sleep apnea can also be inherited from a family member. Congenital malformations and misalignments of the lower jaw can also cause sleep apnea. Individuals who have narrow airways in the throat, mouth, or nose (in this case, mainly due to polyps and nasal septum curvature) will be more prone to suffer from this condition. In young children whose adenoids are enlarged, sleep apnea may also develop gradually. People who smoke, have high blood pressure, are at risk of stroke, or suffer from heart failure have a noticeable increase in their risk of sleep apnea. Excessive alcohol consumption or regular use of sleeping pills also promote this condition.

There are three types of sleep apnea, two of which are far more common than the third type:

1. Obstructive sleep apnea syndrome

By far the most common form is obstructive sleep apnea syndrome (OSAS). The direct cause of OSAS is the -during sleep- almost complete relaxation of the ring-shaped muscles around the upper airways. As a result, the upper part of the trachea can no longer offer enough resistance to the negative pressure created during inhalation. The upper part of the trachea collapses leading to obstruction of the airways.

2. Central sleep apnea syndrome

The second type of sleep apnea is central sleep apnea syndrome. This purely central sleep apnea is rather rare. Due to damage in the central nervous system (CNS), the respiratory muscles are inadequately controlled, and the brain "forgets" to breathe, so to speak. As a result, the respiratory muscles can no longer receive the correct signals from the brain. This in turn causes the oxygen content in the blood to drop, which makes people wake up. Central sleep apnea is usually hereditary, but can also result from neurological damage (e.g., Lyme disease). Individuals suffering from heart failure or heart disease are also much more likely to suffer from this type of sleep apnea.

3. Mixed sleep apnea syndrome

The third type is called complex or mixed sleep apnea syndrome. This is a combination of the other two sleep apnea syndromes already mentioned. Often, obstructive sleep apnea syndrome also triggers central breathing cessations, so the mixed form is also very common.

CHAPTER 3: WHAT SYMPTOMS INDICATE SLEEP APNEA?

The most obvious sign of sleep apnea is loud and continuous snoring. Those affected may well take a short "snoring break". After this "snoring break," however, it often happens that they then suddenly gasp for air. This makes them look as if they are about to suffocate. If they sleep on their back, the snoring becomes even louder. On the other hand, if they sleep on their side, the volume of snoring decreases. Since this state of snoring and wheezing occurs during sleep, they may not know that this is a respiratory problem. Usually, others notice these symptoms and this unusual sleep pattern and let them know about it. By the way, these other people are very important in terms of making a diagnosis for sleep apnea. This will be discussed in more detail in the next chapter. At this point, however, it should be mentioned that chronic snorers do not necessarily have to suffer from sleep apnea. Chronic and loud snoring is an indication, but not a mandatory prerequisite.

The following signs and symptoms, which many people do not associate with sleep apnea, may well indicate it:

a) Headache in the morning

b) Frequent urination in the evening or night hours.

c) Moody behavior up to a conspicuous change in the personality of the affected person

d) Concentration difficulties up to memory loss

e) Dry mouth and dizziness after getting up.

f) Depressed mood

g) Daytime sleepiness up to the tendency to fall asleep

Being overweight or obese increases the risk of suffering from sleep apnea. This is because overweight people have extra-soft fatty tissue. This tissue can thicken in the trachea. The opening of the trachea is not very large anyway, so any further thickening of the tissue leads to a narrowing of the trachea.

Low oxygen levels, or a lack of oxygen in the bedroom, also mean that people are unable to get a restful night's sleep. This is because low oxygen levels cause the muscles of the upper airways to tense up when the trachea is open. In order to relieve this muscle tension, these people begin to snort and gasp for air again before being able to breathe normally. Due to the low oxygen concentration and the accompanying sleep disturbances, more and more stress hormones are released. This can cause these people to be prone to high blood pressure, be at risk for stroke, experience cardiac arrhythmias, and even suffer a heart attack. The stress hormones can also cause them to suffer from heart failure. If this condition is not treated, there is also an increased risk of diabetes.

As one can already see from the previous explanations, sleep apnea or sleep disorders (this will be discussed in more detail in Part II of this book) trigger chain reactions that can lead to much more worrisome diseases. However, this disease progression is not inevitable if a reliable diagnosis for sleep apnea is made in time and the appropriate treatment is initiated. The next chapter will first deal with how such a diagnosis can be made in the first place.

The procedure for establishing a diagnosis for sleep apnea initially involves doctors asking the person affected questions about their medical history. Among other things, this involves determining which symptoms have already manifested themselves in them or previous generations (if known). In some cases, the physician may also ask other family members of the affected person about the extent to which they have observed symptoms, such as chronic snoring. Topics such as the patient's particular sleep patterns are also addressed. After that, doctors have a physical examination. They prepare a report on the symptoms of these people. Then, if they conclude that the signs, symptoms, and patterns of illness point to sleep apnea, these people might be asked to undergo a sleep study. Sleep studies are nothing more than assessments or measurements of sleep patterns. The results show how much and how well they sleep. If patients have any problems with their sleep, the studies will record those results as well. The study can determine if patients are suffering from a sleep disorder, such as sleep apnea. The extent to which sleep studies are useful in terms of diagnosing sleep apnea is going to be the subject of

Chapter 5. The second part of this book is going to deal in detail with the issues surrounding the topic of "sleep disorders".

Sleep apnea and other sleep disorders can increase the health risk for strokes, high blood pressure, and heart attacks. Physicians who have sufficient experience in evaluating sleep studies can quickly determine if individuals are suffering from sleep apnea and then take the appropriate steps to help patients get back to a better night's sleep. The most important thing for patients is to keep their doctor informed about their sleep habits. In particular, they should let their doctor know if they have trouble falling asleep or wake up in the middle of the night and then can't get back to sleep.

People who do not get enough sleep at night will almost always complain of dullness and even chronic fatigue during the day. There are also known cases when people suffer from a sleep disorder without being aware of it. Doctors who specialize in diagnosing sleep disorders are also called sleep *specialists*. These sleep specialists will not find it difficult, based on the symptoms, to diagnose sleep apnea syndrome (if present) fairly quickly and initiate appropriate treatment.

To diagnose sleep apnea, doctors will usually do the following:

1. Keep a sleep diary

Before patients undergo a sleep study, they will usually be asked to complete a so-called "sleep diary" for no less than two weeks. This is the prelude to the sleep study. Here are some questions that the sleep diary is designed to answer:

a) What time did you go to bed last night?

b) What time did you wake up in the morning?

c) How many hours did you sleep last night?

d) How often did you wake up during the night?

e) How long did it take to fall asleep last night?

f) What medications did you take last night?

g) When did you wake up in the morning in case you were still awake in bed when you "went to bed"?

h) When did you wake up in the morning in case you were tired when "going to bed"?

i) How many caffeinated drinks did you have during the day?

j) How many alcoholic beverages did you have during the day?

k) At what time or times did you take the alcoholic beverages?

l) How many "naps" did you take during the day?

m) How long did these "naps" last?

n) Did you feel very sleepy during the day?

o) Did you feel just a little tired during the day?

p) Did you feel wide awake during the day?

q) Did you have a headache in the morning?

r) Did it take you longer than half an hour to fall asleep?

2. Physical examination

During the physical examination, your doctor will primarily check the areas around the throat, nose, and pharynx. He will look for enlarged tissue in these areas. As mentioned earlier, children who suffer from sleep apnea often have enlarged tonsils. This condition alone, along with the medical history of the child, makes it possible to diagnose sleep apnea fairly reliably. When examining adults, on the other hand, doctors will look for an enlarged uvula (also called cervical uvula), which belongs to the soft palate and is located in the middle of the soft palate.

3. Interview family members

Since many people do not even know that they suffer from sleep apnea, there must be someone who notices unusual or abnormal sleep behavior. Many people are usually unaware that their breathing can stop at any time during the night and resume later. Even when confronted with being chronic and loud snorers, it does not raise their suspicions of sleep apnea. There are things family members can do to help:

a) You should let them know that they snore loudly during the night.

b) You should ask them to consult their doctor about this.

c) If the physician diagnoses them with sleep apnea, family members should advise them to follow the instructions, including any follow-up treatments.

d) Family members should also be emotional support for those affected by simply making it clear that they are there for them during this time. After all, this can be a difficult time for those who are affected by this health issue. Therefore, they will need all the support they can get.

CHAPTER 5: TO WHAT EXTENT DO SLEEP STUDIES HELP IN DIAGNOSIS?

Sleep studies are usually performed in a sleep center or a sleep laboratory. Both can be located in a hospital, but this is not mandatory. If the study is done in a sleep lab, individuals will usually spend the night there. Undergoing a sleep study is a painless act. The only thing sufferers complain about from time to time is skin irritation caused by the sensors. However, as soon as the sensors are removed from the skin, the skin irritations subside. Sleep studies usually extend for several hours. Various tests are performed for this purpose. In most cases, patients are first subjected to a **polysomnography test (PSG test)**. In this test, patients have electrodes placed on their scalp, face, chest, and fingers. While they sleep, the following points are monitored and recorded on monitors:

a) The movement of the eyelids

b) Brain activity (brain wave image)

c) The activity in the muscles (muscle tension).

d) The heart rate

e) The heart rhythm

f) The blood pressure

g) The oxygen content in the blood

h) The respiratory movement

i) Breath flow (mouth and nose)

j) Body temperature

The following figure shows an example of the details as well as the measuring points of a polysomnogram:

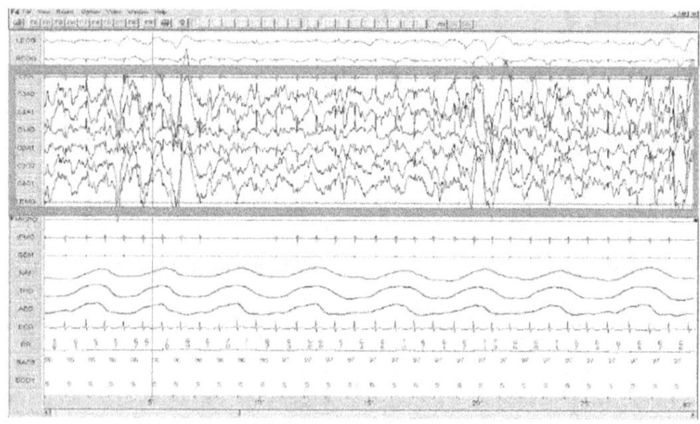

Source: Wikipedia

C3 = top left central

C4 = top right central

A1 = left ear

A2 = right ear

O1 = left occipital (left occiput)

O2 = right occipital (right occiput)

Chin EMG (EMG1 chin left, EMG2 chin right)

LEMG = laryngeal electromyogram (EMG1 larynx left, EMG2 larynx right)

After the PSG test is completed, the results are discussed with the patients. These results allow a reliable prognosis as to whether the patients actually suffer from sleep apnea and whether this condition is already at a worrying stage. Based on these results, the sleep specialist will then be able to initiate appropriate treatment.

To determine how sleepy the patient is during the day, another test is also performed, which is the **Multiple Sleep Latency Test (MSLT)**. This test is usually performed after a PSG test. Similar to the PSG test, the patient is also connected to a meter via multiple electrodes. In this test, patients are asked to take naps of approximately 20 minutes at intervals of 2 hours each. This is repeated at least 5 times, i.e., for at least 10 hours. Once the 20 minutes have elapsed, patients are woken up again by the attending physician. The purpose of this test is to determine how long it takes for patients to fall asleep and how long they sleep. Thus, the test measures the tendency to fall asleep and the duration of sleep. Those who take less than five minutes to fall asleep are suspected of having a sleep disorder during the night due to their high tendency to fall asleep during the day. Once the testing is complete, the sleep specialist will discuss the results with the patient and advise them on treatment options.

The next chapter will discuss the extent to which children can also be affected by sleep apnea, before going on to discuss treatment options in the chapter following the next chapter.

CHAPTER 6: CHILDREN AND SLEEP APNEA

Children diagnosed with sleep apnea use to exhibit strikingly hyperactive behavior, which can even take on aggressive traits. This sleep disorder often leads to a noticeable drop in school performance. They also tend to be bedwetters even at an advanced age. Strikingly, some of them are much more likely to breathe through the mouth rather than the nose during the day. Other signs such as loud snoring, snorting, gasping for air, or temporary cessation of breathing also indicate sleep apnea. The signs and symptoms are similar to those of adults. However, despite these noticeable symptoms, doctors might still not be able to immediately determine that children suffer from sleep apnea. This is because children are usually very active creatures anyway, so doctors will not immediately conclude from their active behavior that this is hyperactivity, which may even be due to a sleep disorder, such as sleep apnea. However, there are some things parents can do to find out if their child is suffering from sleep apnea:

1) See a pediatrician and talk to them about the symptoms parents have observed in their children.

2) Consult an otolaryngologist (ear, nose, and throat specialist) to look at the areas around the nose, mouth, and throat.

3) Parents should also consult a pulmonologist (lung specialist) who specializes in treating children.

4) Psychiatrists and psychologists can also be useful in making a diagnosis.

Parents should be careful to consult physicians who specialize in treating children with sleep apnea. They should also not be afraid to ask about this qualification when filling out credentials. After all, nothing less than their child's health is at stake. The doctor will also ask questions about whether the child is taking any medications and if he or she is allergic to anything. Parents should be proactive in helping the doctor make a diagnosis and let him know of any problems regarding their child's behavior and development. In addition, they should let the physician know about their child's nighttime sleep habits. Finally, the child may undergo a sleep study and, in particular, a PSG test so that a reliable prognosis can be made as to whether he or she suffers from sleep apnea and the severity of the condition. For the effectiveness of sleep studies, please refer to the last chapter.

However, additional tests can be done to make a diagnosis, such as.

1) An electroencephalogram (EEG), which measures brain waves.

2) An electrooculogram (EOG) is used to measure the movements of the retina.

3) An electrocardiogram (ECG), measures heart rhythm and heart rate.

4) Tests to measure the oxygen content of the blood.

The majority of sleep studies will require the child to stay overnight in a sleep lab or sleep center. There are not many medical facilities that specialize in making a diagnosis for sleep apnea in children. From there, parents will often have to visit sleep centers that primarily study sleep disorders in adults. In that case, parents should inquire whether the medical staff also has experience with children who have sleep disorders. Parents should be very selective to find a qualified sleep specialist. Just as in adults, sleep apnea that is left untreated can result in serious health problems in children. In children, it can even have a devastating effect on their behavior patterns and academic performance if not treated in time. If parents notice these changes in their child, they should seriously consider the extent to which a sleep disorder, such as sleep apnea, may be the cause.

CHAPTER 7: WHAT TREATMENT OPTIONS ARE USED FOR SLEEP APNEA?

The treatment of sleep apnea has only one purpose: to enable the patient to breathe regularly again during sleep. However, the treatment also helps to free patients from the annoying habit of loud snoring. A significant decrease in chronic fatigue, which can sometimes last throughout the day, has also been reported after sleep apnea treatment. Finally, therapies that successfully treat sleep apnea also prove beneficial for other health risks, such as heart disease, diabetes, and high blood pressure. There are several options for treating sleep apnea. The following are some of the most common:

1. Lifestyle change

a) People who use to sleep almost exclusively on their backs are significantly more susceptible to sleep apnea. The position in which one lies in bed has an effect on the quality of sleep that should not be underestimated. The position can be responsible not only for the gradual development of sleep apnea but also for its intensity. With people who sleep on their backs, apnea can occur as often as 80 times an hour. Lying on your back causes the tongue and soft palate to be in a recumbent position. And this, in turn, entails blockage of the airways, which strongly promotes repeated cessation of breathing. But this dilemma can be avoided by changing the sleeping position: Sleeping repeatedly on the right or left side, or even on the stomach, will bring noticeable relief. However, this change will not have the desired effect on overweight people.

b) In the case of overweight, weight loss measures should be considered. These people should go for a weight loss plan in consultation with the doctor. A healthy diet, such as fresh fruits and vegetables, is highly recommended.

Physical activity is also highly recommended. It contributes in a special way to the successful treatment of sleep apnea.

c) Sleeping pills and other anesthetics must be avoided at all costs. You should also avoid alcohol as a sedative.

d) The nasal area must not be blocked. If people have problems keeping this clear, the use of a nasal spray should be considered. They may also take decongestants. However, this option is not intended for long-term use.

d) You should sleep with the head elevated to increase oxygenation.

e) Avoid smoking at all costs!

2. CPAP therapy (Continuous Positive Airway Pressure - positive pressure therapy).

If lifestyle changes do not help, there are many indications that it is a serious case of sleep apnea. In such cases, the use of CPAP therapy is very promising. CPAP (Continuous Positive Airway Pressure) therapy is a method that uses CPAP breathing therapy devices. These devices have a blower that is connected via a tube to a CPAP mask that is placed on the face with the use of headgear around the nose (or around the mouth and nose). The use of these masks causes a slight positive pressure of 5-20 millibars to be created in the airways during sleep. This slight air pressure helps keep the passages of the upper airways open, preventing airway collapse and thus sleep apnea. This therapy is also referred to as "pneumatic splinting" of the upper airway. When using these therapy devices, a significant decrease in loud snoring can also be noticed.

However, the use of these masks (a distinction is made in this context between "direct nasal," "oral," "nasal," and "full-face masks") takes some time to get used to. This is because counterpressure is regularly generated during exhalation, which requires a certain amount of effort from the patient - at least in the initial phase. As a rule, CPAP respiratory therapy devices are set to the individually required ventilation pressure in the sleep laboratory. This pressure can be checked in sleep laboratories and adjusted at regular intervals, as it can change in the course of therapy, such as when a patient loses or gains weight.

If the appropriate adjustments are made to the headgear that is placed on the face, people can get used to wearing these masks more quickly. Patients can ask their doctor or a sleep specialist how to make the appropriate adjustments. In addition, a humidifier can also provide additional comfort along with the CPAP breathing therapy device. However, you should not let this "uncomfortable" feeling at the beginning of this treatment slow down your decision to seriously consider this therapy. After all, after a period of acclimatization, most users report significantly improved sleep quality and even a decrease or disappearance of sleep apnea. Discontinuing the therapy can cause symptoms to return. In order to benefit from this therapy, it is critical to implement it regularly.

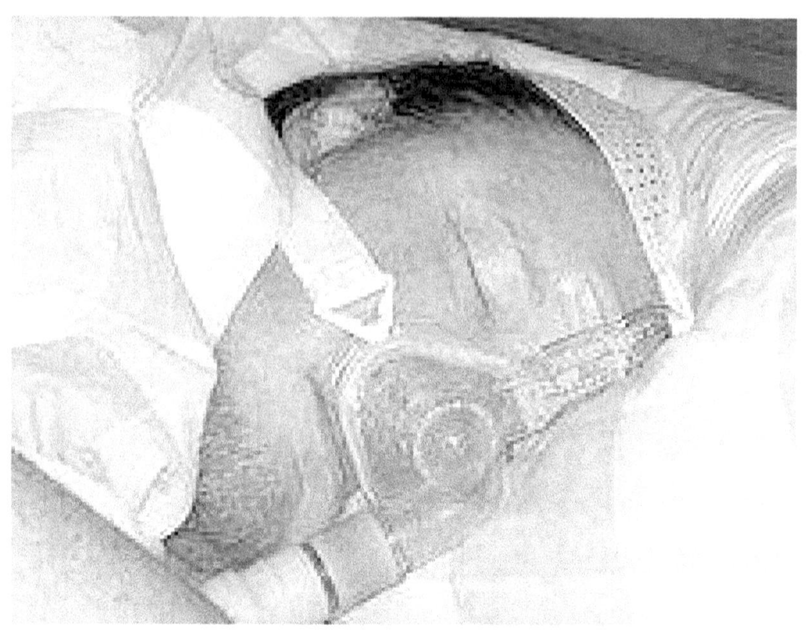

User with CPAP mask (source: Wikipedia)

Nevertheless, some of the side effects when using CPAP therapy should also be briefly mentioned:

a) Eye irritation

b) Counterpressure during exhalation

c) Upper respiratory tract infections if the respirator is not kept clean.

d) Irritation of the nasal mucosa

e) Pain in the mouth

f) Dry mouth

g) Discomfort of the chest muscles

Conclusion: CPAP therapy is both a highly effective and most commonly used therapy to treat sleep apnea. However, it is a symptom-treating therapy. It does not cure the disease.

3. Intraoral Protrusion Device

How does the intraoral protrusion device work?

The intraoral protrusion device is supposed to hold the lower jaw and the tongue in position to prevent breathing pauses during sleep. This device must always be tailored-made for the person suffering from sleep apnea. It is a two-position adjustable device that needs to be worn in the mouth during sleep. This way, the lower jaw, and tongue are held further forward, keeping the muscles stable and the airway open. Since the throat muscles slacken and the tongue sinks back during sleep, which promotes sleep apnea, the intraoral protrusion device uses to prevent that. As a result, there are significantly fewer breathing pauses. Treating patients with the intraoral protrusion device is a very effective measure to prevent sleep apnea.

4. Surgical intervention

Surgery is another option that may be considered to treat sleep apnea. Unlike CPAP therapy, a surgical procedure is used to pursue a cure for this condition. During such a procedure, excess tissue is removed from the nose or throat. This procedure is performed only in a hospital. Another way of treatment is to reduce or stiffen the excess tissue. Patients are given medication before the surgery so that they can sleep. Therefore, during the operation, they will not be aware of the surgical procedure. After the operation is performed, patients often complain of a sore throat for about 7 to 14 days afterward.

Generally, the following surgeries are considered for sleep apnea:

a) UPPP (Uvulopalatopharyngoplasty) surgery.

This is a procedure in which tissue is removed from both the back and front of the throat. In addition, the palate and tonsils are also removed. This surgery may succeed in stopping snoring during the night. However, since there is still tissue in the throat, it is unlikely that sleep apnea can be successfully treated with this surgery. The remaining tissue causes insufficient oxygen to be transported through the trachea. UPPP surgery is only performed in a hospital. So, the patient needs to be treated in a hospital for this procedure.

At this point, I would like to point out that this operation is very painful. Patients who have undergone this surgical procedure might need several weeks to recover. This surgery is performed only in patients who suffer from severe obstructive sleep apnea. However, even in these cases, few opt for this surgery. So, UPPP surgery does not belong to the category of those surgeries where you can get up and go back to business as usual shortly after. The following complications may occur during UPPP surgery:

1) Irritation in the area of the soft palate and neck muscles.

2) Sore throat if no antibiotic was taken before surgery.

3) Difficulty swallowing

4) Ingested liquids may leak back out through the mouth or nose.

5) Impairment of the sense of smell

Despite this painful operation and its side effects, there is no guarantee that patients will sleep significantly better afterward. Even after the operation, they may still experience periods when they suffer from sleep apnea.

b) Tracheotomy - surgery

However, some surgeries can be performed orally. Tracheotomy surgery is usually performed only when previous treatments have failed. It is generally only considered when the sleep apnea syndrome has already reached life-threatening proportions. In this surgery, a metal or plastic tube is inserted through an opening in the throat to help patients breathe. This opening remains closed during the day and is only opened again at night.

c) Bimaxillary surgery

During this operation, the breathing space behind the tongue is enlarged. For this purpose, the upper and lower jaws are moved forward. This increases the oxygen concentration in the arterial blood. Since this procedure is complex, it is not uncommon for an oral surgeon and an orthodontist to work together in performing this breathing space augmentation. Surgeons use laser technology to remove additional tissue in the throat to enlarge the breathing space. The use of radiofrequency energy is also common. Both procedures also promise the long-term elimination of snoring.

In a study conducted in 2008, the researcher found out that 93.3% of patients who underwent this surgery reported a good to even excellent quality of life afterward: Widening the nasopharynx had an extraordinarily positive effect on general productivity, social success, overall activity, alertness, concentration, and sexuality. In contrast to UPPP surgery, the surgical risks associated with bimaxillary surgery are low: surgery was unsuccessful in only 4 of 177 patients.

5. Sleep apnea pillow

Given that some people who sleep enough (at least 7-8 hours) still feel tired after getting up is still an issue that needs to be addressed more carefully. This may be related to nocturnal snoring. At this point, it should be noted that snoring is a very serious medical problem. To address the problem of "snoring", sleep apnea pillows have proven to be very useful for some people. However, before chronic snorers reach for a sleep apnea pillow, it should be made sure whether their case is exclusively a "snoring problem" or whether the snoring is a result of sleep apnea. However, even in the case that sleep apnea is not the cause of snoring, sleep apnea pillows can help reduce snoring. Sleep apnea pillows can help reopen or keep open blocked airways. This is because sleep apnea leads to irregular and repeatedly interrupted breathing. Sleep apnea pillows are used to restore regular breathing. The irregular and interrupted breathing usually happens during the night when they are sleeping. These special pillows are made of foam and have a slight elevation, unlike regular pillows. The elevation serves to keep the head in an "inclined" position, which should allow for even and uninterrupted breathing. Sleep apnea pillows can also be adjusted individually. This allows them to be used in a way that provides the most sleep comfort for the patent. They can significantly help to regain restful sleep during the night.

Unfortunately, too few chronic snorers still use this type of pillow. They rather prefer to take sleeping pills and eventually become dependent on them. Medication is not a good alternative to successfully treating snoring or sleep apnea. There is much to suggest that medication has proven ineffective in combating these conditions.

Let us sum up the most important things discussed:

1) Sleep apnea is a chronic condition that causes sleep to be repeatedly interrupted during the night by cessations or cessations of breathing.

2) Since snoring is considered by many people to be something completely normal, this condition often remains undetected for a long time. At this point, however, it should be mentioned that chronic snorers do not necessarily have to suffer from sleep apnea. Only sleep studies, which chronic snorers should undergo, provide clear information about this issue.

3) Among the three sleep apnea syndromes (obstructive, central, and mixed), obstructive sleep apnea occurs most frequently.

4) As a result of sleep apnea, chronic sleepiness can develop during the day, which can lead to industrial accidents or other injuries.

5) Overweight people who suffer from sleep apnea should take weight-reducing measures. Medical advice and help should be sought in this case.

6) Family members should talk to those people suffering from cessations of breathing if they notice

their loved ones repeatedly gasp for air during the night. The later this condition is detected, the greater the likelihood that it will result in even more serious illnesses. This is because people who suffer from sleep apnea tend to have high blood pressure. So, they are at risk of stroke, use to frequently suffer from cardiac arrhythmias, and may even suffer a heart attack.

7) In children who exhibit behavioral problems and whose performance in school drops sharply, this circumstance is not usually associated with sleep apnea. For this reason, parents should carefully observe their children, especially during sleep, to determine whether their behavioral problems and drop in performance may not be due to sleep apnea.

8) Others should also not make fun of those who suffer from sleep apnea. Sleep apnea is a very serious sleep disorder that should be treated with urgency.

Depending on the severity of the condition, the doctor or sleep physician will devise a suitable treatment plan to effectively treat sleep apnea.

If you have ever suffered from insomnia, you are probably aware of how much this condition drains your energy and life quality. Insomnia weakens and debilitates the body. It is a terrible feeling to never get enough sleep and to toss and turn in bed all night. People who suffer from insomnia are unable to get the rest at night that the body needs to face the challenges of the next day. This can have disastrous effects on nearly every aspect of life. According to a report by the U.S. Department of Health and Social Services, approximately 64 million Americans suffer from insomnia. Research studies found that women are 1.4 times more likely to be affected by insomnia during their lifetime than men. In Germany, about 20% -30% complain of sleep disorders. In the second part of this book, the term "insomnia" is first examined in more detail. Then, some of its causes will be analyzed and effective ways to effectively combat sleep disorders will be shown. Once you have also read the second part of this book, you will have a much better understanding of sleep disorders and will be able to take the appropriate steps necessary to solve this problem. This is because, in order to be able to treat the condition of insomnia, you must first gain a clear understanding of this condition. One must study the causes of it and its consequences, that is, how insomnia eventually affects the body.

First, let's start with what insomnia is in the first place: insomnia is not just tossing and turning in bed during the night because you can't fall asleep. It's also not a phenomenon that happens only occasionally. Every person has "bad" sleep at night now and then. Often this is the case if the brain has not yet fully processed the impulses of the day and therefore much of it happens during the night. This is quite a normal process that should not be categorized as "insomnia.", Insomnia is rather the inability to <u>regularly</u> find restful sleep because one is no longer able to sleep through several hours. The German Society for Sleep Research and Sleep Medicine writes on this subject: "*There is no binding temporal norm for the amount of sleep required to ensure restfulness. Most people know the amount of sleep from their own experience.*" So, it can be inferred in reverse that sleep - regardless of the duration of sleep - which permanently no longer causes recovery, indicates a possible disorder. This lack of sleep leads to physical and mental fatigue during the day and affects all areas of life.

CHAPTER 2: SLEEP DISORDERS, SLEEP PATTERNS, AND SYMPTOMS

Sleep disorders often have the following symptoms:

a) Migraine and headache

b) Lack of concentration

c) Waking up several times during the night

d) Constant signs of fatigue

e) Memory lapses up to memory loss

f) Slight irritability

Although there are different degrees of sleep disorders, three types of sleep disorders can be distinguished:

1. Temporary insomnia

A temporary sleep disorder can last from a few days to several weeks. It can be triggered by stress, depression, changes in the sleep environment, or another illness.

2. Acute insomnia

Acute insomnia is diagnosed when this condition lasts for at least three weeks and up to 6 months.

3. Chronic insomnia

Physicians use to diagnose chronic insomnia when this condition lasts continuously for the whole year or even for several years. Chronic insomnia is often the consequence of another disease. However, this is not necessarily the case, i.e. chronic insomnia can also be the primary disease.

Before getting to the bottom of the actual causes of sleep disorders and taking appropriate treatment measures, it is important to assign the condition to one of these three categories mentioned. In the next chapter, we are going to analyze these causes and treatment measures in more detail.

Sleep disorders often have two distinct <u>sleep patterns:</u>

1. Difficulty falling asleep

Some people - and regardless of whether they are tired or not - cannot fall asleep after lying down in bed. Interestingly, people who feel very tired also experience this condition. However, as soon as they go to bed, they are suddenly wide awake again.

2. Sleeping disorders

Some people can fall asleep effortlessly, but wake up in the middle of the night and then can't get back to sleep.

Or they wake up too early in the morning and then can't fall back asleep either.

Scientists have now intensively studied what happens to the body during sleep. In the process, they have repeatedly concluded that sleep is vital. Sleep deprivation not only significantly impairs quality of life, but can often be a catalyst for other very serious health issues. Sleep is enormously curative for both physical and emotional overload. Sleep restores the body's functions and resets the internal clock to zero. For those who suffer from insomnia, the internal clock continues to run uninterrupted, so that collapse is virtually pre-programmed. We know that we need rest. The body's message is unmistakable but our mind often ignores this message.

Against this background, the following metabolic process takes place in the body: Cortisol is a hormone that activates metabolic processes and thus provides the body with energy-rich compounds. It also tells the brain when it is time to relax and prepare for sleep. This hormone usually follows a 24-hour cycle, making us feel awake in the morning hours and relax in the evening. This hormone keeps us active, alert, and creative during the day. In the evening, the release of this hormone slows down and cortisol levels begin to drop to prepare the body for sleep during the night. As a rule, the human body has its lowest cortisol level about 3 ½ hours after sunset. People who suffer from insomnia have a different, higher level of cortisol. This hormone level is thus no longer in its natural balance, which also leads to an impairment of the natural sleep rhythm. Even though the German Society for Sleep Research and Sleep Medicine has no guideline for the length of sleep that ensures restful sleep, you should go for a sleep duration of seven to eight hours. It is highly recommended to go to sleep at 22:00 or 23:00 at the latest. This is because the following principle has proven to be effective: *One hour of sleep before midnight is better than two hours of sleep after midnight.*

It has been scientifically proved that sleeping strengthens the immune system. In addition, sleeping is crucial for the regeneration of cells and tissue in the organs. This regeneration process usually requires about five hours. However, unfortunately, people who suffer from insomnia usually sleep significantly less than five hours.

It is a feeling of powerlessness to have to drag yourself through the day completely overtired and exhausted due to sleepless nights and not being able to do anything about it. Moreover, this miserable feeling can also lead to a dramatic end: Insomnia, if left untreated long enough, can lead to death. Our bodies need rest like the air we breathe. Rest is therefore not just something we can consider desirable or optional. Sleeping is not a "luxury item" that we can simply do without compromising our quality of life. Rest is essential to life. Just as bodybuilders need to allow their muscles to rest after an intense training phase (because muscles always develop in the resting phase, not the active phase), we too need to allow our minds and bodies to relax after a stressful and challenging day. And this complete recovery is only achieved by sleep. If people suffer from sleep disorders for a long time, they will reach a point where all mental and physical functions will "shut down" and stop working.

With this in mind, there can be no doubt that insomnia is a very serious problem and that those affected by it must be prepared to do something about it. Unfortunately, reading this book and being aware of the seriousness of this health issue will not solve the problem. Knowledge of this disorder is an essential part of your efforts to eliminate it. However, this knowledge will not bear fruit unless you put it into practice.

After the different types of insomnia, the different sleep patterns, and the symptoms have been discussed in this chapter, the next chapter will deal with the causes of this disorder. People who suffer from insomnia will probably identify with some of these causes. I would like to ask you to write them down on a piece of paper. Do not trust your memory regarding this very important subject. Because if you are suffering from insomnia, it may not be working in the way you want it to. You will need this information later.

CHAPTER 3: CAUSES OF AND REMEDIES FOR SLEEP DISORDERS

The following causes are often associated with sleep disorders:

1. Stress

Stress is a phenomenon that has reached unprecedented levels in today's world of hustle and bustle. As a result, the body is continuously under pressure. Less time is devoted to rest. Today's motto seems to be as follows: Those who are constantly busy and under stress are considered to be in demand and important. Stress seems to have become an indicator of important people. Of course, this is not necessarily so. Given that around 10% of CEOs surveyed suffer from burn-out syndrome may underline this assumption.

Stress can and will have devastating effects on health if not counteracted in time. People who are constantly under stress are no longer able to relax completely. This is particularly noticeable in a gradually increasing sleep disorder. Because to fall asleep, complete relaxation is a basic prerequisite. If this prerequisite is not met, one will long for a restful sleep in vain. At this point, however, it is necessary to check very carefully whether stress is really the cause of a sleep disorder or whether it is insomnia itself that is causing the stress. So here it is a question of which came first, the chicken or the egg. For further treatment, however, it is very important to be able to answer this question for oneself or with the help of others.

Of course, every person suffers from stress at some point in his or her life. This is inevitable and a normal experience. Relationship problems, health concerns, and financial difficulties can put a lot of pressure on our lives, creating stress. With this in mind, the important question to ask is how to deal with stress. Workouts, massage baths, social contacts, a balanced diet, and a positive attitude might not be able to eliminate stressful situations but will significantly reduce their outflow on our physical, mental, and spiritual life.

It may also be that stress results from situations that have their origins in the past. In that case, it is crucial to target these problems - also with the help of therapeutic support - to solve them or let them go. Solving these problems can have a great impact on the quality of sleep. The step into the past is often painful. However, if it is taken and the "disposal" of these issues is successful, it will have a tremendous health impact not only on the present but also on that person's future. As a result, you might be rewarded with a significant increase in the quality of sleep.

Stress can also be due to financial difficulties. This type of stress seems to increase dramatically given the current situation in the world. Financially stressful situations require, among other things, the preparation of a monthly budget, competent debt counseling, and the help and support of family members and friends. Make also sure to ask for the help of a reputable and reliable financial advisor. These people are trained to set up customized financial plans by identifying redundant expenses. Talk to friends and family members about the problem. They often look at things more objectively and alert you to things you may not realize yourself. Take a proactive approach to manage this problem. It's often hard to look at your behaviors from an objective point of view. This is even more true if you seem constantly tired and exhausted due to existing sleep disorders.

As mentioned earlier, stress is one of the most common triggers for insomnia. It can have a devastating effect on health. Insomnia, as well as many other diseases, is an indication that the body is no longer in balance. So, it is essential to find out which areas of your life are out of balance. You may notice that insomnia caused by stress will disappear as soon as these areas of your life are brought back into balance.

2. Room temperature

Surprisingly, sleep disorders are very rarely connected to room temperature. However, if the bedroom is too hot or too cold, it affects the quality of sleep. People who suffer from sleeping disorders should ensure that the room temperature is at a "comfortable" temperature for sleep. The optimal temperature for sleeping is 62 -66°F. Besides, you should also make sure that the room temperature does not change constantly during the night because the body reacts to temperature differences very sensitively, which causes a wake-up reaction if the bedroom should become too hot or cold.

3. Room lighting

Both the room temperature and room lighting are often underestimated when it comes to sleep disorders. So, it is important to ensure that those who suffer from sleep disorders are in a room that is as dark as possible. Darkroom conditions are optimal for the production of the sleep hormone melatonin. Make sure to pull down the blinds before going to bed so that you are not awakened too early in the morning by daylight. This is especially true in the spring and summer months when it gets light very early. If blinds are not available, a sleep mask will also help. Put this on before you go to sleep. This allows you to create a darkening effect at any time, regardless of the lighting conditions inside or outside the bedroom, which significantly promotes falling asleep.

4. Diet

A balanced diet is also important for restful sleep. Sleep disorders can also be caused by an unbalanced diet. Time and again, it has been shown that many diseases can be successfully treated by changing dietary habits. However, special attention should be paid more to the *timing of* food intake than to the diet itself. People who eat hearty meals before bedtime make their bodies stay awake so they can perform their function of burning calories again. This leads to an increase in cortisol levels and thus turning the body's sleep mode off. This is because cortisol is a hormone that activates metabolic processes providing energy to the body. However, when this energy is provided at night or late in the evening, it can significantly inhibit sleep.

Since caffeinated beverages are known to stimulate circulation, it goes without saying that people who suffer from insomnia should definitely avoid them in the evening. In this context, it has been proven as a guideline not to take caffeinated beverages after 4:00 pm.

5. Snoring

As already discussed in detail in the first part of this book, snoring is often an indication of sleep apnea. Snoring can be causative of this sleep disorder. Snoring is usually considered very annoying by those who try to sleep next to a loud snorer. Many patients were very surprised when after a sleep study they were told by sleep specialists that it was their snoring that made them wake up and caused the sleep disorder. This should not be surprising, considering that many snorers are not even aware that they are snoring at all. Therefore, in order to correct the sleep disorder in such cases, the cause (snoring) must be eliminated. At this point, I would like to refer to part I of this book, in which various therapeutic options related to sleep apnea and snoring had been discussed.

6. Working time

People who have to work various shifts due to their profession are much more exposed to sleep disorders than others who have a "normal" workday. Professionals who repeatedly have night shifts and then try to sleep during the day experience that it is much more difficult for the body to shut down all functions during the day to induce sleep. The reason why is that the aforementioned hormone cortisol keeps us active, awake, and creative during the day. It is only in the evening that the release of this hormone slows down, and cortisol levels begin to drop. The release of the sleep hormone melatonin requires darkroom conditions. As discussed earlier, it is possible to artificially induce darkening, such as by pulling down blinds or putting on sleep masks. However, unfortunately, our minds cannot be completely convinced that it is night again during bright daylight.

7. Age

With increasing age, the metabolic processes in the body also change. As a result, sleep-promoting processes are no longer carried out in the same way in old age as in younger years due to the decrease in the production of the sleep hormone melatonin resulting in difficulties falling asleep and staying asleep. In such cases, melatonin tablets can prove very useful. Since this is a natural sleep hormone, no harmful effects are usually to be expected. Nevertheless, medical advice should be sought in this case as well.

8. Diseases

In case the sleep disorder still exists even after all the causes mentioned have been eliminated, the sleep disorder is likely to organic or neurological disease. The following diseases use to lead to a significant impairment of sleep quality and thus to a serious sleep disorder:

a) Respiratory diseases

As mentioned in the first part of this book, pathological respiratory arrests lasting longer than ten seconds cause the oxygen content of the blood to drop (hypoxemia). This leads to a deficiency in the supply of oxygen to the tissues and, as a result, there is an awakening reaction in the body. A sufficient amount of oxygen, which the body obtains through the air, is therefore essential for a relaxed night's sleep. Anything that impairs oxygen intake via the lungs also disturbs sleep. In addition to sleep apnea, these can include a stuffy nose from a cold, sinusitis, bronchitis, pneumonia, or bronchial asthma. Acute lung disease or bronchial asthma can also cause life-threatening shortness of breath. These asthma attacks lead to considerable difficulties in falling asleep and sleeping through the night.

In cases where the sleep disorder is due to respiratory disease, anti-inflammatory, and bronchodilator drugs for inhalation, tablets for sucking or swallowing, heat applications or, if necessary, hyposensitization treatment may be considered, depending on the underlying diseases mentioned. If the underlying disease is due to bacterial inflammation, treatment is by the use of antibiotics. In any case, the patient should consult his or her physician, who will first listen to the lungs and examine the nasopharynx before referring the patient to an ear, nose, and throat specialist or even an allergist.

b) Cardiovascular diseases

Given that people who suffer from sleep apnea are prone to high blood pressure, can have heart failure (cardiac insufficiency), and can even succumb to a heart attack. However, there is not only a causal relationship because these diseases mentioned (high blood pressure, heart failure, heart attack) can themselves trigger a sleep disorder, i.e. they can also be the cause and not only the result of a sleep disorder. To prepare the body for sleep, the heartbeat slows down and blood pressure begins to drop. Any awakening, whether conscious or unconscious, such as a cessation of breathing, causes the heart rate to increase and blood pressure to rise again. This up and down leads to a strong strain on the heart function, causing the release of stress hormones that can dramatically disturb the night's rest.

If cardiovascular disease is suspected, patients should always consult their physician. He or she will examine blood pressure, listen to the heart, and perform an electrocardiogram (ECG). If the suspicion of a cardiac arrhythmia, a heart defect, or heart failure is confirmed, a long-term ECG, blood tests, and an ultrasound examination of the heart may also follow. If the suspicion of cardiovascular disease is subsequently confirmed, medication or therapeutic measures are taken, such as bypass or bypass surgery or the insertion of a pacemaker.

However, to prevent this from happening, a healthy lifestyle must be pursued at all costs. At this point, successful stress management, a balanced diet, and regular physical activity should be pursued regularly.

c) Heartburn

Heartburn occurs when stomach acid flows back into the esophagus, causing a painful burning sensation in the stomach. If coughing fits occur more frequently in the early morning hours, this is an additional indication of this condition. This painful reflux of stomach acid into the esophagus can also lead to a dramatic disturbance of the night's rest.

If you should suffer from these symptoms, you should consult your physician, who may do further tests, such as laboratory tests. In addition, a referral to a gastroenterologist, i.e. a specialist in gastrointestinal diseases, might be recommended. He or she will then decide whether a gastroscopy and other examinations should be performed.

In this case, a balanced diet, relaxation, and successful stress management are the keys to getting this problem under control. If these measures do not result in heartburn gradually subsiding, you should ask your physician to check whether the **Helicobacter pylori** bacterium is responsible for the pain. If this is the case, the use of an appropriate antibiotic will quickly provide relief. This bacterium is repeatedly responsible for gastritis and stomach ulcers.

Please take my advice in this context: You should explicitly tell your doctor to check for the presence of this bacterium. In my family, relatives suffered from massive stomach pains for several years without a doctor having identified this bacterium as being responsible. After these relatives had specifically asked the doctor about this and their suspicion had been proven to be true, an appropriate antibiotic was used immediately for treatment. As a result, the stomach pain disappeared within a short time.

With this in mind, I want you to be spared these unnecessary very painful years by simply being proactive when visiting your doctor.

d) Joint and muscle diseases

In principle, all diseases that cause pain disturb sleep. This is especially true for joint and muscle diseases: Back pain, muscle tension, chronic joint diseases such as arthritis, wear and tear diseases of the joints (osteoarthritis), tendonitis, and tumors in bones and joints can be very troublesome sleep disruptors. People can already be prevented from falling asleep by joint and muscle pain if the diseased joint moves into an unfavorable position when lying down. This can also lead to an awakening reaction of the body after falling asleep and thus also disturb sleep.

Suspicion of a joint or muscle disease should be discussed with your physician. He will initiate the appropriate investigations and, as in the case of arthritis, recommend anti-inflammatory medication. At this point, however, it should be pointed out that some medications used to treat inflammatory joint diseases unfortunately also carry the risk of triggering sleep disorders themselves. For this reason, it should be ensured in consultation with your doctor that a chain reaction is not triggered as a result.

e) Hyperthyroidism

Hormones have a decisive influence on the quality of sleep. Hormonal fluctuations and hormonal disorders, therefore, lead to a dramatic impairment of sleep quality. The thyroid gland plays a decisive role in hormonal control. It produces essential hormones in the body, which are indispensable for many processes in the organism. In this context, it has a decisive impact on the central nervous system, the cardiovascular system, digestion, the psyche, and much more. If the thyroid gland is out of balance, hormonal fluctuations are inevitable. In the case of hyperthyroidism, the thyroid gland produces too many thyroid hormones. Against this background, sleep disorders are a typical indication of hyperthyroidism.

If hyperthyroidism is suspected, your physician will perform a blood test as a first step. This may be followed by further examinations, such as ultrasound scans or thyroid scintigraphy. The treatment of a thyroid disorder is usually carried out with the help of medication. They are intended to bring hormonal fluctuations back into balance. Afterward, people that had been affected by this will be able to sleep better again.

So, this chapter has focused on five diseases that can cause sleep disorders. By the way, this is not a conclusive enumeration. Therefore, other diseases, such as neurological diseases, can also be the cause of a sleep disorder. The extent to which a sleep disorder can be attributed to another disease should therefore be discussed with a physician. However, the diseases discussed are particularly often associated with sleep disorders. For this reason, they have been given special attention in this chapter.

61

The second part of this book focused on the different types of sleep disorders (transient, acute, chronic), the different sleep patterns associated with sleep disorders (falling asleep and staying asleep), and their symptoms. After that, possible causes of sleep disorders were discussed in detail, as well as ways to remedy them. It turned out that sleep disorders can only be eliminated if their actual cause has been determined. Against this background, sleep studies conducted in a sleep center by sleep specialists are very helpful. Acute and chronic sleep disorders must be treated. Delaying therapy can have a disastrous effect on physical, mental, and emotional well-being. Even small lifestyle changes, such as room temperature suitable for sleep, dark lighting conditions, or a balanced diet, can significantly reduce a sleep disorder. Sometimes it takes greater effort, such as successful stress management, which sometimes requires taking a step back in time or seeking outside professional advice to get this problem under control. Those who are willing to be proactive in solving this problem will be rewarded with finding restful sleep again and thus achieving the quality of life that many had never dreamed possible.

Congrats! Note from the Author:

You've reached the end of the book!

Thank you for finishing **THE SLEEP EASY SOLUTION BOOK!**

Looks like you enjoyed it!

If so, would you mind taking 30 seconds to leave a quick review?

It would mean the **WORLD** to me!

I work hard to bring you books that you enjoy!

Plus, it helps and encourages me dramatically to produce more books like this in the future!

www.ingramcontent.com/pod-product-compliance
Lightning Source LLC
Chambersburg PA
CBHW061715130726
47996CB00006B/2315